MW01244900

THE FOOD ALLERGY HANDBOOK

A Practical Guidebook

Melissa Cole

ISBN-13: 979-8-39-551170-6

Cover design by: Melissa Cole
Cover Artwork by: Jaime Pike
Library of Congress Control Number: 2018675309
Printed in the United States of America

This book is dedicated to my children
Jonathan, Annemarie, Jaxon
and my husband, Jon.

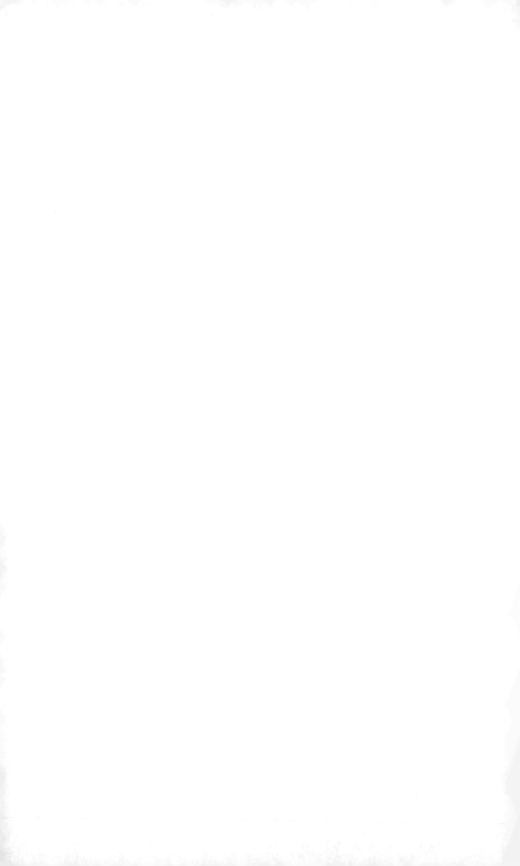

CONTENTS

CHAPTER ONE

HOW IT BEGAN

Twenty-seven missed calls.

I scrolled through my text messages. There were too many to count. The calls were all from my son's daycare, my husband, and my Mom.

Why is the daycare calling so many times? Something is wrong.

Two days prior, I traveled to another state for business meetings. After lunch on this fateful day, I placed my phone in my purse on vibrate. The time for our mid-afternoon break was approaching, so I just checked my phone while the speaker wrapped up. Instantly, as I saw the notifications on my phone, my gut screamed that something terrible must have just happened. I called my husband and he wasn't answering his phone. The calls from the daycare meant something was wrong with my one-year old son, whose birthday was this very day. Panic set in...*what has happened*? I tried to call my Mom. No answer. My heart was racing. My mind was going to terrible places. The fear was so intense, it felt as if I was being smothered. The feeling of helplessness was overpowering. I listened to my voicemails. My entire world started crumbling at my feet. *Something was wrong with my baby!*

The voicemail from my husband told me my youngest son

was in trouble. My husband did not know what exactly was happening to him. His voice was panicked.

Finally, in what felt like years but was only about 2 minutes, my husband called me back and explained everything. The daycare decided to have a "special day" and offer the kids peanut butter and jelly sandwiches for lunch, though they were normally peanut-free. My sweet one-year old boy immediately began having a severe allergic reaction, *on his first birthday.*

My Mom, who rushed to the daycare, did not recognize him when she got there due to his face swelling to the point he was beyond recognition. If it wasn't for his bright red hair, she would not have known that swollen boy was her grandson. Our world was rocked that day, as it is for many food allergy families with their child's first reaction. Thankfully, the day care and my mother responded quickly, and his reaction subsided with prompt treatment.

After the conversation with my husband, I learned my son was already treated and recovering fine. Thank the Lord for that! The panic turned instantly to guilt. *I should've been there.* I'm his Mama and he needed me. I tried to imagine how he felt. His face, mouth, and throat were swelling, tingling, and itching. Anxiety must have set in as his symptoms began to intensify. He began having trouble breathing and felt strange, out of sorts. How horrible my sweet baby must've felt. Seeing the fear in those around him must have intensified his own feelings. In my heart, at this moment, I told myself that I would never leave his side.

So, I took an earlier flight home and cried my eyes out on the plane. My poor baby. I can't begin to describe the millions of thoughts that went through my mind. I was never leaving him again. I was quitting my job. He would never be in daycare ever again. The food pantry would be cleared out of all peanut contaminated food the instant I got home. Peanuts are stupid little things! I was never letting him go...

Tears poured and poured. Thank God for window seats. I imagine I felt almost as alone on that plane as my son did earlier that day.

We had no idea, until that first reaction occurred, that he had any food allergies. Once he was tested, we discovered he had allergies to peanut, egg, dairy, tree nuts, corn, and wheat. My son's first allergic reaction to food changed our lives. It's one of those moments in life that I will remember clearly forever, as is the first time I administered an epi-pen in my son's leg. That distinct look of fear in his eyes is something that evokes sadness just from recalling the event. The carefree days of eating out at restaurants, attending birthday parties anxiety-free, and grocery shopping met an abrupt end that day.

Life changes immediately for all members of a food allergy family. Our entire home was reassessed for food safety. Handwashing is our new obsession. No sharing drinks or food anymore due to fear of cross contamination. We learned to read food labels *like it's our job.* Carrying an EpiPen Jr is more important than carrying my wallet. My other children tell strangers not to feed their little brother **anything**. Life changes drastically.

Fellow #FoodAllergyParents

Constant protection, Epi-Pens, and Benadryl. Always on alert for danger and ready to react swiftly. This is the daily experience of a parent with a child with life-threatening food allergies.

Fear and anxious anticipation can drown your trusting heart in a matter of seconds when a severe allergic reaction starts. It becomes hard to shake the anxiety that comes with keeping your child safe. Balancing safety and normalcy becomes a new skill. Keeping your child included and safe becomes your cross to bear. Not many will understand how a food allergy family lives differently. There will be judgement, exclusion, and sorrow at times. But there is hope. We are not alone in this fight for survival. Studies reveal that one in thirteen children in the United States has a food allergy. The world will have to learn how to deal with this growing issue.

As parents, we are charged with encouraging and forcing the world make a place for our children to live and grow up safely. When a child receives a severe food allergy diagnosis, it feels like the world stands still for just a moment while you try to figure out what to do next. I remember the doctor handing me my son's lab report after his first reaction and saying something like, "You'll need to avoid these foods. We will recheck in a year to see if anything has changed."

I remember holding that lab report in my hand and thinking it was completely useless. *Avoid these foods...really? I kind of figured that much, thanks. That's all you're going to tell me? Isn't there a book or something you could give me? So, what can I feed him? Should he go back to daycare or is it unsafe? Should my family eliminate these foods in our home? Should I find another doctor, a specialist? Are there other families going through this and how do they cope?*

Five million questions came to mind, and I had the answers to none of them! Along the bumpy path that has been my involuntary commitment to the food allergy odyssey, I have learned the answers to the questions I had on that first day and the days following. In the following chapters, allow me to share the tools, resources, and information that I wish I had when this journey started. Let's share in this expedition and make the world a safer place together.

◆ ◆ ◆

DEVOTION

"Where no counsel is, the people fall: but in the multitude of counselors there is safety." Proverbs 11:14 King James Version

With support, our difficult journeys become easier. With encouragement, we can face each struggle with confidence. With each other, food allergy sufferers and their families, we find strength & resilience that others cannot understand. Draw on the strength of the Lord and the friends he places on your path, and your burden will become lighter, easier to bear.

Prayer: Dear Lord, surround me with encouragers, lift me up in your strength. Help me on this journey to find and lean on the counselors you have placed on my path. Help me to then become a counselor to others. In Jesus' Holy name I pray, Amen.

CHAPTER TWO

WHERE TO START

F ood allergies are an immune response to a substance that your body mistakenly thinks is a threat. The body overreacts to the food allergen, with the most severe reaction leading to anaphylaxis, which can lead to death. Epinephrine auto injectors can stop the anaphylactic response. The top eight food allergens, meaning the most common, are eggs, milk, peanuts, tree nuts, fish, shellfish, wheat, and soy. Sesame is not currently included in the top eight but there is debate that it should be for required labeling purposes.

- Do you have the right doctor?

Once your child receives a diagnosis of a food allergy, your first step should be to determine if you have the best doctor for the diagnosis. There are a lot of allergy doctors around but not so many that specialize in food allergies. My son first received his diagnosis from an Ear, Nose, and Throat specialist that also treated seasonal type allergies. Once he had his first reaction, the pediatrician referred us to the allergist in town. Food allergies were certainly not his specialty as evidenced by how we were handed the lab report that listed his allergens and told to avoid those foods. That was it. No guidance. No direction.

We went almost a year before finding a true food allergy specialist at the Children's Hospital in our state, after a friend whose son also had food allergies urged us for months to make the switch. After our first visit with the specialist, we felt tremendously better about how we were handling our son's food allergies. The fog seemed to lift from the world of uncertainty and doubt we had grown accustomed to. The specialist explained a lot about food allergies and how our son's food allergies might change over time. The specialist was supportive and encouraging. As parents, we needed that validation that we were taking good care of our son. We also needed the information the specialist and nutritionist shared with us to feel more confident in our decisions.

I wish we had sought out a specialist that was dedicated to food allergies sooner. We may could have saved ourselves a lot of stress by becoming more informed sooner. As a food allergy parent, you cannot always rely on the advice or encouragement of well-meaning friends or family. They simply don't understand how to approach food allergies, unless of course they have a child with food allergies themselves.

After you find your food allergy specialist and have a few appointments, don't be afraid to switch if you are not happy with them. Trust your gut. There are specialists that do no keep up with the latest research and may not serve your child at the level necessary. When our family found a revolutionary food allergy treatment program, our food allergy specialist had never even heard of it. I was shocked because it has been around awhile and people from other countries fly in just to be in the program. No one is more motivated than you as a parent to seek out cutting edge information and treatments, not even food allergy doctors.

- Ground Zero: Rebuilding a food list & eliminating hidden food allergens (list of tricky ingredient names)

The best way to start with building a safe food list is beginning at ground zero. Think about all the foods that are safe and can be added. Usually, whole & clean foods are an easy place to start. The more processed a food is, the more risk of unsafe ingredients and cross contamination. Foods that never see a factory are usually the safest- fresh meats, vegetables, fruits. The fewer ingredients, the better.

Depending on your child's specific food allergies, you will want to become familiar with hidden allergen ingredient names. The FARE website (foodallergy.org) is a great resource to start learning those tricky ingredient names. Always be aware that warning labels such as "may contain" and "processed in a facility that also processes ____" are voluntary and therefore, not regulated or checked by any regulatory agencies.

- EpiPen Jr-Always carry at least 2 and store them properly

Whatever your preferred epinephrine auto-injector brand may be, always carry two of them. One dose may not be enough. An auto-injector may malfunction so always have a backup. At one time, epi pen jrs were recalled for this very reason. Be sure to check your packaging and keep the auto-injectors at the specified temperature, as they lose effectiveness if they are in high temperatures.

Many manufacturers offer coupon codes to reduce the cost of copays on auto-injectors. They can get quite costly, especially when you want to have multiple sets on hand, such as keeping a set at home, one for daycare, and one for travel. Take advantage of the coupons.

- Unsafe foods and what to do with them in your home

Our family quickly came to the conclusion that we needed to clean out our food supply, getting rid of most of the food our son was allergic to. This was very difficult at first and we held on to a few things because it was so hard to break our own food habits. Our son was allergic to peanuts, tree nuts, dairy, egg, wheat and corn. Many of these foods were staples around our house. When he was first diagnosed at one year old, it was easier to control the food he consumed. As he grew older, it was more and more difficult. We put a child proof lock on our food pantry. Our older children made keeping our food allergic son safe more challenging, as they were already accustomed to eating dairy in multiple forms, eggs for breakfast and peanut butter regularly. My oldest son loved peanut butter and jelly sandwiches and ate one for lunch quite often. It became too stressful for us to have his allergens in the house so we eliminated all peanut products and rarely had dairy and egg in the house. Thankfully, his allergies to tree nuts, wheat and corn disappeared by age 3. Interestingly, corn is one of his favorite foods now.

On one occasion, we had cow's milk in the house and I was making the older kids chocolate milk. I had also poured Jaxon's soy milk in a cup and sat it in a separate place on the island in our kitchen. I walked across the kitchen to get a spoon to stir the chocolate syrup into the cow's milk and while my back was turned, my food allergic son took the cow's milk and drank it, thinking it was his soy milk. That was the first time we had to use the epi pen on him ourselves. It was the scariest thing I've had to do as a parent. Injecting a shot seems so simple until you have to do it in a stressful moment that is already filled with fear and panic. My son was screaming so hard, he wasn't making any noise. My husband held him down while I injected the epi-pen jr. I didn't even get it in the right spot on his leg but it did work. We rushed to the hospital where he was given more meds and observed for several hours. Thank God he was ok.

◆ ◆ ◆

APPLE SLICED CAKE RECIPE

This cake is one of my husband's all-time favorites from when he was a child. I adapted it so my son could also enjoy it!

1 ¾ cup sugar

1 cup oil

Egg substitute= 3 whole eggs (I use Bob's Red Mill Egg Substitute)

2 cups organic flour

1 cup chopped walnuts (free of cross contamination with peanuts, other tree nuts)

2 cups organic apples sliced thin and cut in half

¼ cup organic applesauce, unsweetened

1 teaspoon baking soda

1 teaspoon organic cinnamon

1 teaspoon salt

1 teaspoon good quality vanilla

Preheat oven to 350 degrees. Prepare egg substitute according to directions. Beat sugar, oil, and egg substitute. Add dry ingredients, vanilla and applesauce. Mix well. Add apples and nuts and stir in. Pour into a greased glass casserole pan. Bake at 350 degrees for 40-60 minutes. Cool and enjoy!

CHAPTER THREE

LABELS

In 2006, "top eight" allergen labeling became mandated by the United States Food and Drug Administration in all packaged foods manufactured and marketed in the US. The top eight food allergens are milk, egg, fish, shellfish, tree nuts, wheat, peanuts and soybeans. At that time it became easier for consumers to identify what packaged foods contained their allergens.

The ingredients must be listed on the packaging and also identified at the end of the ingredient list as a "Contains" statement, i.e. "Contains: Milk, Egg."

Many packages also include a "May Contain" statement. This statement is placed on the package to alert consumers that the product may contain food allergens by cross contamination, though it may not be an ingredient in the product. This cross contamination occurs when production lines and equipment are shared with other products made at the same facility. They may produce a product such as a cookie that does not contain peanuts in it's ingredients, but earlier have produced a peanut butter cracker on the same equipment, thereby creating cross contamination.

The utterly terrifying aspect of "May Contain" statements is that they are completely **VOLUNTARY**. While I am thankful to the companies that include these alerts, I'm frightened by the products of companies that do not include these cautionary statements. It only takes one tiny peanut protein to incite anaphylaxis in my son. A word of caution to those with food allergies (and the parents of children with food allergies): call the company that produces the products to ensure there is no chance of cross contamination if they do not label with "may contain" statements. If you must be strict on cross contamination, I'd advise you to utlilize this step in asessing the safety of the food prior to consuming, especially for new products.

Always check food labels, as sometimes ingredients change. Some companies, such as Chick-fil-a, will notify you of ingredient changes but not all companies do this. Double check, even if it's a tried and true safe product for you.

While the US has come a long way in product labeling, we still have more work to do in full disclosure regarding packaged food products. My prayer is that "May Contain" labeling becomes mandatory very soon. Be aware and be safe.

◆ ◆ ◆

THE BEST CHOCOLATE CHIP COOKIE RECIPE

(Allergy friendly to nut, dairy and egg allergies)

The first time I made these cookies, my food allergic son wouldn't touch them, but the entire family loved them and gobbled them up. My son was so scared to try new things. It took much reassurance that they were safe before he would try one. Now he loves them! We make a huge cookie-cake for his birthday from this recipe! I've also made this recipe for my son's preschool class. All of the 3-year-olds (and the teacher) loved it.

¾ cup refined coconut oil, melted (refined to eliminate coconut flavor)

¾ cup packed brown sugar

¾ cup granulated sugar

½ cup applesauce

1 ½-2 teaspoons good quality vanilla

2 ½ cups all-purpose flour (preferably unbleached)

1 teaspoon baking soda

½ teaspoon baking powder

1 teaspoon salt

¾ cup dairy-free chocolate chips (I use Enjoy Life brand)

Preheat oven to 350 degrees Fahrenheit. Prepare the baking sheet with cooking spray, parchment paper or silicone cookie pan liner. Using a stand mixer with paddle attachment, combine the coconut oil, sugars, applesauce and vanilla until smooth. In a separate, medium bowl, combine the flour, baking soda, baking powder and salt with a wire whisk. Add the flour mixture to the wet mixture and stir until combined. Stir in the chocolate chips.

Using a cookie scooper, place the batter onto the prepared baking sheet. You may want to smoosh the cookie batter down with a spatula for a flat cookie. Bake for 12 to 15 minutes, or until lightly browned. Cool completely before serving. Enjoy!

CHAPTER FOUR

EDUCATING YOURSELF ON ALL THINGS FOOD ALLERGY

A s the days passed, my family and I began to adjust to our new life with food allergies. We quickly realized that this was not a temporary condition, and we needed to adapt and make some significant changes to our lifestyle to keep our son safe.

We started by educating ourselves on food allergies and reading about the various types of food that could trigger an allergic reaction. We learned about cross-contamination and how even the tiniest trace of an allergen could cause a severe reaction. We became experts in reading food labels and quickly learned how to identify hidden allergens in processed foods.

The first few weeks were challenging, but we slowly found our rhythm. We began to understand the importance of always being prepared and carrying our son's EpiPen and Benadryl with us at all times. We also became skilled in managing social situations, such as birthday parties and playdates. We would always bring our son's food with us and let the other parents know about his allergies.

We found a community of other parents with food-allergic children, and this was a significant source of support and comfort for us. We were all in the same boat, and it was reassuring to know that we were not alone. We exchanged tips and advice on managing different situations and shared our experiences and fears.

Despite the challenges, our son's food allergies brought our family closer together. We learned to appreciate the little things and cherish the moments we spent together. We also found creative ways to make food fun and enjoyable for our son, who had to follow a restricted diet. We experimented with different recipes and discovered new foods that he could eat.

Living with food allergies is not easy, but it has taught us some valuable lessons. We have learned to be more empathetic and compassionate towards others who may be dealing with different challenges in their lives. We have also become advocates for food allergy awareness and are committed to raising awareness and educating others about the dangers of food allergies.

Looking back, I realize how much our lives have changed since that fateful day when my son had his first allergic reaction. But, in many ways, it has changed for the better. We have learned to live in the moment, appreciate the little things, and never take anything for granted. We are grateful for every day that we have together and feel blessed to be a part of a community of strong and supportive food allergy families.

- Educate yourself (resources)
  1. Food Allergy Research & Education (FARE) - A non-

profit organization that offers information on food allergies, including resources for families, education programs for schools and communities, and advocacy efforts to improve food allergy policies.

2. Allergy & Asthma Network - Provides educational resources for food allergy sufferers, including information on managing allergies, finding allergy-friendly restaurants, and understanding food labeling.

3. The Asthma and Allergy Foundation of America (AAFA) - Offers resources for managing food allergies, including tips for navigating social situations and traveling with allergies, as well as advocacy efforts to improve food allergy policies.

4. American Academy of Allergy, Asthma & Immunology (AAAAI) - Provides resources for patients and healthcare professionals, including guidelines for managing food allergies and a directory of allergists.

5. Kids with Food Allergies Foundation - Offers resources for families with children who have food allergies, including recipes, tips for managing allergies in school, and a support community.

6. National Institute of Allergy and Infectious Diseases (NIAID) - Provides information on food allergies, including research updates, clinical trials, and guidelines for managing allergies.

7. Food Allergy and Anaphylaxis Connection Team (FAACT) - Provides resources for families and individuals with food allergies, including education, support groups, and advocacy efforts.

8. Allergic Living - A magazine and online resource that provides news, information, and advice for people with food allergies and sensitivities.

9. Food Allergy Canada - A non-profit organization that provides resources for Canadians with food allergies, including information on managing allergies in school, traveling with allergies, and finding allergy-friendly products.

10. AllergyEats - An online guide to allergy-friendly restaurants, with user-generated ratings and reviews from people with food allergies.

Don't be afraid to educate your medical team. They are teaching you about the medical condition and you are teaching them about the patient. It's essential to ensure that your child's medical team is aware of their food allergies. Here are some steps you can take to educate your child's medical team:

1. Compile a list of your child's food allergies and keep it with you at all times. You can create a simple document that lists all the foods your child is allergic to, the symptoms they experience when exposed to those foods, and the appropriate treatment.

2. Make sure your child's medical records reflect their food allergies. This information should be included in your child's medical history and should be readily available to any healthcare provider involved in their care. Don't forget the dentist, as some dental products have been found to contain dairy.

3. When meeting with a new healthcare provider, make sure to inform them of your child's food allergies. You can provide them with a copy of the list of food allergies you've compiled and explain the importance of avoiding those foods.

4. Ask your child's healthcare provider to provide you with a written action plan that outlines what steps to take in case of an allergic reaction. This plan should include clear instructions on what medications to administer, when to seek emergency care, and how to prevent future reactions.

5. Consider working with an allergist or immunologist to help manage your child's food allergies. These specialists can provide valuable insight into your child's condition, develop a comprehensive treatment plan, and help you educate your child's medical team on the best practices for managing food allergies.

By taking these steps, you can help ensure that your child's medical team is aware of their food allergies and is equipped to manage any allergic reactions that may occur. Remember, education is key, and the more you can inform your child's medical team, the better prepared they will be to provide the best possible care.

One form that can be used to compile information on a patient's food allergies and treatment is the Food Allergy & Anaphylaxis Emergency Care Plan developed by Food Allergy Research & Education (FARE). This form is designed to be completed by the patient's healthcare provider and includes important information such as the patient's food allergies, symptoms of an allergic reaction, emergency contact information, and treatment instructions.

The form can be downloaded for free from FARE's website in both English and Spanish, and can be customized with the patient's specific information. In addition to the emergency care plan, FARE also provides other resources such as a food allergy action plan, food allergy & anaphylaxis emergency care plan for schools, and resources for healthcare professionals. I place this form in my child's emergency medical bag.

If you have a child with food allergies, it's important to educate their siblings on how to keep them safe. Here are some steps you can take to educate your other children:

1. Explain the severity of the food allergy: Sit down with your other children and explain what a food allergy is and how severe it can be. Make sure they understand that their sibling could have a life-threatening reaction if they eat the wrong food.

2. Identify the allergen(s): Teach your other children which foods their sibling is allergic to and what they need to avoid. Make sure they know how to read food labels and understand cross-contamination.

3. Teach them to recognize symptoms: Teach your other children to recognize the symptoms of an allergic reaction, such as hives, difficulty breathing, or vomiting. Explain that if they see their sibling experiencing these symptoms, they need to get an adult immediately.

4. Encourage handwashing: Make sure your other children understand the importance of washing their hands before and after eating. This can help prevent cross-contamination.

5. Practice empathy: Teach your other children to be empathetic towards their sibling with food allergies. Encourage them to be supportive and understanding if their sibling can't eat certain foods or needs to take extra precautions. Using analgies the child will understand can help them to be more empathetic.

The same strategies can be applied for educating your family, church, and your child's school. Unfortunately, the burden lies on you to educate all spheres of your child's world but would you want anyone else to be responsible for it? The more people can understand your child's condition, the better equipped they are to help them stay safe.

It's important to find a support group that meets your specific needs and offers the resources and support you need to manage your food allergies. Here are some food allergy support groups that can be helpful for individuals with food allergies, as well as parents of children with food allergies:

1. Food Allergy Research & Education (FARE): FARE is a nonprofit organization that provides education, advocacy, and support for individuals with food allergies and their families. FARE also hosts a variety of events and programs for individuals with food allergies.

2. Allergy and Asthma Network: The Allergy and Asthma Network is a nonprofit organization that provides education and support for individuals with allergies and asthma. They offer a variety of resources and support groups for individuals with food allergies and their families.

3. Kids With Food Allergies (KFA): KFA is a division of the Asthma and Allergy Foundation of America (AAFA). KFA provides education, support, and advocacy for families of children with food allergies. They offer a variety of resources, including online forums and support groups.

4. Food Allergy Kids of Atlanta: Food Allergy Kids of Atlanta is a nonprofit organization that provides education and support for families of children with food allergies. They offer support groups, educational events, and advocacy programs.

5. No Nuts Moms Group: No Nuts Moms Group is a Facebook group with over 25,000 members. The group provides support and resources for moms of children

with food allergies. They offer a variety of resources, including recipes, tips for dining out, and product recommendations.

6. Spokin: Spokin is a mobile app that provides resources and support for individuals with food allergies. The app includes a directory of allergen-free restaurants, product recommendations, and a community forum where users can connect with other individuals with food allergies.

♦ ♦ ♦

DEVOTION

"What do you think? If a man has a hundred sheep, and one of them has gone astray, does he not leave the ninety-nine on the mountains and go in search of the one that went astray? And if he finds it, truly I say to you, he rejoices over it more than over the ninety-nine that never went astray. So it is not the will of my Father who is in heaven that one of these little ones should perish." Matthew 18:12-14

It can be a lonely place dealing with food allergies. Many will not support or understand your challenges. But don't give up hope just yet! There are people that care, that want to help. Cherish them, thank them, return their kindness every chance you get. There are angels that were once bound by food allergies that are now free from that pain and are watching over us. Food allergy kids are resilient. They live through tough days and still smile. They appreciate small acts of kindness with more depth than many. When so many people ignore their plight, the one that shows concern erases away the ones that don't. It's the kind of "special" one feels when Jesus leaves the 99 to recover you, the one lost sheep.

Prayer: Dear Lord, Give my child resilience in their fight against food allergies. Help us as parents to make good decisions and be on alert for their safety at all times. Help us watch over them. Open our eyes to the ones that show kindness and make our children feel special. Show us ways to spread kindness. In Jesus' Holy name I pray, Amen.

CHAPTER FIVE

ALLERGEN EXPOSURE

I magine you walk into a room at one of your favorite places, maybe a restaurant in which you've enjoyed many meals or a park at which you've spent many afternoons daydreaming. You notice that this time your favorite place is different. Something feels off...it feels dangerous. You look around trying to identify what is different. You can't tell at first but soon you start to see it...a minefield of explosives.

Most people would run in the other direction. You'd have to be crazy to walk into a minefield, right?

Yet, this is exactly what those with food allergies face every time they go to a public place. A minefield.

Now, imagine that it's not you walking into your favorite place that is now so extremely dangerous...*but it's your child.* Your sweet, innocent child that is not prepared to identify dangerous situations as an adult would.

Think of this place as a park with a playground. What was once a place to have fun and "be a kid" is now filled with explosives for your food allergic child. Innocent, unaware children are walking around eating a PB&J sandwich, wiping it off their face and then touching the slide that your child is about to go down. Never-mind that there is a picnic table nearby, the parent isn't paying attention and the child is roaming around eating. Another child is running around with their sippy cup of milk, dripping it on the playground equipment. Your child has a life-threatening allergy to all of these foods that are now all over the playground. This place is no longer fun. It is dangerous.

Do you steal your child's experiences of "being a kid" to keep them safe? Do you take them to the minefield and hope for the best? How do you handle this situation? It's one that food allergy families face daily.

Until you come face to face with the fact that the same food that is considered healthy for some will in fact kill your child, you might not be able to imagine the dangers present in everyday life.

Until you've had to witness your child struggle to breath, scratch their tongue vigorously with both hands, look into your eyes with a primal fear, vomit and go limp....all from one bite or drink of the wrong food, you might not understand why it's so important to prevent exposure. Until you've feared that one epi-pen jr isn't enough to stop the anaphylactic response in your child, you might not understand why it's so important to prevent exposure. Until the hospital nurse has told you they have called the chaplain to come speak to you, you might not understand why it's so important to prevent exposure.

Let me explain this clearly: it is CRUCIAL to prevent exposure.

Each anaphylactic response can become more rapid and deadly with each occurrence. It's as if the body's response gets stronger each time. The best way to prevent quicker, stronger anaphylaxis is to avoid exposure altogether. It's not as simple as just giving an epi-pen. Sometimes they don't work. Sometimes it's too late to stop the anaphylactic shock. Sometimes the child does not see the other side of anaphylaxis. It is a sobering truth that many need to hear.

Our family has experienced several exposures over the years. Our son has accidentally had cow's milk instead of soy milk as a result of me having poured all 3 kids milks in the same looking cups. My son grabbed the wrong one. Lesson learned that day to always use specific, different looking cups for our food allergic son.

Once our son drank from his sister's water bottle by accident, after she had eaten Cheetos. We had no idea he had done this until after he started looking pale and vomiting. After looking around to find out what he'd gotten into, we figured it out. Again, lesson learned and we started using a sharpie marker and writing names on every plastic bottle of water we opened. He was young in both of these instances but as he grew older, he became more and more hesitant to eat or drink without double checking first to be sure it was safe for him.

As a parent of a food-allergic child, it's important to be aware of situations where accidental allergen exposure may occur. We had several experiences when we were out in public or on vacation where contact exposures occurred and caused major issues. We began to wipe everything with disinfecting wipes to be sure there were no residual food proteins on surfaces. Here are some situations where you might not know there has been an allergen exposure and how to handle them:

1. When eating out: It is important to inform the restaurant staff about your child's food allergies and ask them about the ingredients in the dishes you plan to order. However, even with the best intentions, there is always a chance of cross-contamination. If you suspect that your child has been exposed to an allergen, watch for symptoms such as hives, difficulty breathing, and vomiting. If symptoms occur, use an epinephrine auto-injector and call 911 immediately.

2. During playdates: It's important to inform other parents about your child's food allergies before your child attends a playdate. However, it's possible that a well-meaning parent might not realize that a food item contains an allergen. Make sure to pack safe snacks and remind your child not to share

food with their friends.

3. At school: If your child attends school, it's important to work with the school staff to create a plan to keep your child safe. This includes providing the school with a list of your child's allergens, making sure the school has a supply of epinephrine auto-injectors, and ensuring that your child knows not to share food with their classmates.

4. When traveling: Traveling can be particularly challenging for food-allergic individuals. Before traveling, research the destination and food options, and pack safe snacks. Additionally, it's important to inform the airline or hotel staff about your child's food allergies and ask for accommodations such as a special meal or a refrigerator in the hotel room.

In all of these situations, it's important to remain vigilant and prepared for possible allergen exposure. Have an action plan in place in case of accidental exposure and communicate with your child's doctor to ensure that they are receiving appropriate care.

Recognize, React, Give And Go

The phrase "recognize, react, give and go" is a simple way to remember the steps to take when a severe allergic reaction occurs, also known as anaphylaxis. Remembering and following these steps can help increase the chances of a positive outcome in the event of a severe allergic reaction.

- Recognize: This step involves being able to recognize the signs and symptoms of an allergic reaction. These can include hives, itching, swelling, difficulty breathing, coughing, vomiting, or diarrhea. It's important to note that symptoms can vary from person to person, and may not always be the same with each reaction.

- React: Once an allergic reaction is recognized, it's important to react quickly. This may involve administering an epinephrine auto-injector (such as an EpiPen) if one is available. It's important to know how to use the auto-injector and to keep one with you at all times if you or your child has a known food allergy.

- Give: After administering the epinephrine, it's important to give other medications as needed, such as antihistamines or bronchodilators, and to call for emergency medical assistance.

- Go: Once emergency medical assistance has been contacted, it's important to go to the hospital or emergency room for further evaluation and treatment.

Another important term to understand is a biphasic reaction, which refers to a type of allergic reaction that can occur in some people who have experienced a previous allergic reaction. It is characterized by a recurrence of symptoms after an initial improvement, usually within hours or days after the first reaction.

The first phase of the reaction occurs immediately after exposure to the allergen and can range from mild symptoms such as hives and itching to severe symptoms such as anaphylaxis. During the second phase, the symptoms return or worsen even though the allergen has been removed from the body. This second phase can occur without any further exposure to the allergen and may be more severe than the first phase.

Biphasic reactions are considered dangerous because they can occur unpredictably and may not respond to standard treatment for an allergic reaction. In some cases, the second phase of the reaction can be more severe than the initial reaction and may require more aggressive treatment, including hospitalization and intensive care.

Therefore, it is essential for individuals with a history of severe allergic reactions to recognize the symptoms of anaphylaxis, seek immediate medical attention, and be monitored for several hours after an allergic reaction. This is to ensure that they do not develop biphasic reactions or other complications. Furthermore, it is recommended that patients carry an epinephrine auto-injector at all times and know how to use it in case of an emergency. As a good rule of thumb, if you have to use an epipen, go to the hospital. They will monitor your recovery and look out for signs of a biphasic reation.

◆ ◆ ◆

DEVOTION

"Love your neighbor as yourself." Matthew 22:39

Food allergies have become a punchline to some, a weapon to bullies and death to it's victims. More concern, love and sympathy for each other would make all of our burdens easier to bear. And maybe just a little safer for those who need to be loved and protected.

Prayer: Dear Lord, May I always remember your directive to love others and support them in whatever their trial may be. I pray that my child will be protected from his food allergies and will see your love through others that take the time to learn how to keep him safe. In Jesus name I pray, Amen.

CHAPTER SIX

INCLUSION, NOT EXCLUSION

N othing breaks your mama heart more than to see your child feel like an outsider or outcast, especially at an event that is supposed to be a celebration. Ice cream and pizza parties at school, birthday parties, holiday meals-they can all be opportunities for your child to feel excluded because of their food allergies. There are ways to combat that outcome if you spend a little time planning and communicating. Here are some strategies to consider:

1. Communicate with the activity organizer: Before your child participates in an activity, make sure to speak with the organizer about your child's food allergies. Let them know what your child is allergic to and what steps need to be taken to keep them safe.

2. Pack safe snacks and meals: If your child will be away from home during meal or snack time, pack safe snacks and meals for them to eat. Make sure to label them clearly with your child's name and the type of food inside.

3. Educate your child on their food allergies: It's important to teach your child about their food allergies and how to recognize the signs of an allergic reaction. Make sure they know what foods they need to avoid and how to ask questions

about the ingredients in their food.

4. Always carry emergency medication: Make sure to always carry your child's emergency medication, such as an EpiPen, with you. This is especially important during activities that are far from medical help or where it may take some time to get help in case of an emergency.

5. Choose activities wisely: When selecting activities for your child, consider the level of risk for exposure to allergens. Activities that involve food, such as cooking or baking, may be more risky, so make sure to take extra precautions in these situations.

Holidays can take a food allergy sufferer and their family to a whole new level of anxiety. A time that is meant to be joyous and festive is wrapped in fear, trepidation and discomfort for food allergy families. For us, food centered gatherings are no time to relax and enjoy the company of friends and loved ones. Our focus must always be on safety, protection and prevention. Children, teenagers and adults lose their lives at gatherings such as these, even when they do absolutely everything right. There are too many moving parts to a family food-centered gathering, too many variables, too many figurative and actual hands in the pot, too much for us to monitor and ensure safety.

What defines many people's ideas of the perfect holiday may not center around food such as pecan pie, peanut butter cookies, pumpkin pie with whipped topping, candied pecans, cheese balls rolled in nuts, and green beans with sliced & roasted almonds, but it is certainly a major part of their idea of the perfect holiday. We are still fighting to show that one child's favorite lunch food, a PB&J sandwich, is not worth losing the life of another child. Holidays are a whole new ballgame.

If I could embody food allergy sufferers and their families with one trait, it would be perseverance. We keep going, keep advocating, keep protecting, and yes, even keep loving despite all the hurtful, harmful and hateful opposition. Despite all the negative comments, the abandoned friendships, the shunning of family members that just don't get it, we keep going. We persevere.

Keep in mind at this years' family gatherings that we don't want to be a pain or offensive by asking millions of questions about food prep, ingredients, labels, what you ate before you came and other weird-seeming questions to non-food allergy folks. We want to be protected. We want to leave the party in the same car we arrived in, not an ambulance.

For some families, possible exposure is too big a risk to take, especially when the allergy is severe. Please know that we want more than anything to be there. We sacrifice our desires & preferences to keep our children, or ourselves, safe. We ask for no judgement on this decision. I promise it is a painful decision for us to make.

Be careful, my dear food allergy friends. It's a minefield out there. My prayer for you is discernment on what is a safe situation and what is not safe, and of course to always be safe.

My prayer for all non-food allergy friends & families is for understanding, respect and love towards food allergy sufferers. That's the best holiday gift you could ever give us.

◆ ◆ ◆

Recipe

Here's a simple recipe for dairy-free hot chocolate.

Ingredients:

- 2 cups of non-dairy milk (almond, soy, oat, coconut, etc.)
- 2 tablespoons of cocoa powder
- 2 tablespoons of sugar or sweetener of your choice
- 1/4 teaspoon of vanilla extract (optional)

Instructions:

1. In a small saucepan, heat the non-dairy milk over medium heat until it comes to a simmer.

2. Whisk in the cocoa powder and sugar until completely combined.

3. Reduce heat to low and continue whisking until the mixture is smooth and heated through.

4. Remove from heat and stir in vanilla extract (if using).

5. Pour into mugs and enjoy!

Optional toppings:

- Dairy-free whipped cream
- Mini marshmallows (make sure they are dairy-free)
- Cinnamon or nutmeg sprinkled on top

CHAPTER SEVEN

THE EMOTIONAL SIDE OF FOOD ALLERGIES

Food allergies isolate children and their families. That's the truth. It's painful, difficult and defeating all in the same moment. Those are pretty powerful emotions for a child or adult to feel in one concentrated burst, often daily. Children with food allergies have a difficult time participating in all the activities that other children take for granted. Fun childhood experiences like trick or treating, birthday parties, summer camps, Easter egg hunts, Vacation Bible School, and pizza parties at school are not carefree fun for children with food allergies.

They always have to be on alert, keeping their guard up for whatever their poison is: peanuts, tree nuts, dairy, egg, soy, fish, shellfish, wheat and a myriad of other foods.

Be aware that what is an American classic treat, *ice cream*, could be death for some. We consider our allergens poison because we know they can kill us. It's hard to get excited about an ice cream party when ice cream is your worst nightmare. Seeing your siblings get excited to have the food that could kill you is a lonely place to be.

And it's not just the person with food allergies that feels isolated. It's the entire family. It's the Mom or Dad of a food allergy child that has to be persistent and aggressive to keep her/his child safe, often to the point of losing friends or being shunned because we are a little "crazy about food allergies." It's also the brother or sister of a food allergy child that unfortunately has to skip events, sacrificially, because it's not safe for the entire family. Who wants to leave their sibling behind, sad and left out, while you go enjoy the party? It's also the grandparents that have to constantly be alert when their food allergic grandchild is around, upsetting some because of the restrictions that must be in place for the child. Traditions sometimes have to be broken: "Sorry, can't have boiled peanuts this year at our gathering!"

There is a constant, underlying level of anxiety present when you have food allergies. Social norms are not the norm for us. We are different. We are mocked. We are bullied. We are talked about. How could you not have anxiety when the same food that the world is in love with could kill you? The same food that parties are planned around causes a violent reaction in your body with just a trace. You give up so much that others take for granted. There's no denying the loneliness of food allergies. So many people just don't understand and don't even care to.

Creating a safe environment for allowing these emotions to be dealt with is crucial to keep yourself and your child emotionally healthy. As parents, we focus on the physical safety of child on a 24/7 basis. Mental health is equally important. Having safe people to talk to is so important. There is a bounty of online resources, support groups, and counselors that can be that safe space for you and/or your child. You will form bonds and give and receive support in these places that is not as freely given anywhere else.

One thing I've learned over the years of dealing with food allergies it that all of the family has needs related to mental/emotional health. Be sure to spend one on one time with your other children, making them feel focused on as well. Parents need support too. Don't be afraid to seek out mental health services if needed.

◆ ◆ ◆

RECIPE

Here's a recipe for dairy-free snow cream:

Ingredients:

- 8-10 cups of fresh snow

- 1/2 cup of sugar

- 1 teaspoon of vanilla extract

- 1 can of coconut milk (13.5 oz)

- Optional toppings: sprinkles, chocolate chips, fruit, etc.

Instructions:

1. Gather clean, fresh snow in a large mixing bowl. Make sure the snow is clean and free of any debris.

2. In a separate bowl, mix together the sugar, vanilla extract, and coconut milk until well combined.

3. Slowly pour the coconut milk mixture over the snow, stirring continuously, until the mixture reaches a creamy consistency.

4. Continue to add more snow or coconut milk as needed until the mixture reaches the desired consistency.

5. Serve immediately, topped with any desired toppings.

Enjoy your delicious dairy-free snow cream!

CHAPTER EIGHT

KEEPING CURRENT
Food allergy breakthroughs

I t is an exciting time in food allergy research. Researchers are discovering new information daily in the fight against food allergies. Several treatments are now available to food allergy sufferers that have never been available in years past. Oral Immunotherapy (OIT), Tolerance Induction Program (TIP), and Palforzia are all viable treatments for various food allergies. Learning the differences, desired outcomes, success rate, and commitment expectations for each of these will determine your child's best option.

Palforzia was not yet FDA approved at the time of writing this book, however it is very close to becoming the first FDA approved drug for the treatment of peanut allergy. OIT is a medical treatment provided by an allergist that includes a long term solution for a variety of food allergies. TIP is a data analytics approach that utilizes a different methodology than OIT, called protein matching, to desensitize the body to a food allergen. My son is enrolled in the TIP program, only offered at Southern California Food Allergy Institute, now simply known as the Food Allergy Institute. He was on a waitlist for nearly a year in order to enter this revolutionary program that is helping thousands of patients achieve total food freedom. As they have expanded their program, the wait to join the program is much shorter than when we enrolled.

Testing is a good way to diagnose food allergies. There are blood tests and skin prick tests and when the results are used in tandom to diagnose, the accuracy is better. Results can change over time, so your doctor may recommend testing every year or two. Some children do outgrow allergies, meaning they develop the antibodies needed to subdue reactions. Food challenges may be recommened based on lab tests to see if you can tolerate certain foods. We have done many food challenges for my son. Many have gone very well and some have not gone so well. It's important to communicate with your doctor regarding your comfort level with proceeding with food challenges.

Rencently, there have been several treatment advances in food allergy treatment. Here are a few examples:

1. Oral Immunotherapy (OIT): OIT is a treatment that involves consuming small amounts of the allergen in gradually increasing doses over time. The goal of OIT is to desensitize the patient to the allergen and reduce the risk of an allergic reaction. Recent studies have shown that OIT can be effective in treating peanut and other food allergies.

2. Sublingual Immunotherapy (SLIT): SLIT is similar to OIT, but instead of consuming the allergen, the patient is given drops of the allergen extract under the tongue. SLIT has shown promise in treating peanut, tree nut, and grass pollen allergies.

3. Epicutaneous Immunotherapy (EPIT): EPIT is a new treatment that involves applying a patch containing the allergen to the skin. The patch delivers a small amount of the allergen to the immune system over time. EPIT has shown promise in treating peanut allergies.

4. Monoclonal Antibody Therapy: Monoclonal antibody therapy involves giving the patient an injection of an antibody that blocks the immune system's response to the allergen. This

treatment has shown promise in treating peanut and other food allergies.

5. Chinese Herbal Medicine: Some recent studies have suggested that Chinese herbal medicine may be effective in treating food allergies. However, more research is needed to confirm these findings.

It's important to note that these treatments are still in the early stages of development and are not yet widely available. Patients should consult with their healthcare providers to determine the best course of treatment for their individual needs.

Our family chose to start treatment in 2020 at the Southern California Food Allergy Institute. This has been the best decision in our son's food allergy care by leaps and bounds. They treat ALL food allergies in children at the FAI and this has been a life changing program for us. Our son is now safely eating all of his multiple food allergens on a daily basis, in large amounts. He has already cleared dairy and is enjoying ice cream and yogurt daily. I can't express the joy in my heart when he ate his first Oreo Blizzard with our family at Dairy Queen. He loved it and was so excited to share the same treats with his siblings. We are nearing the end of the program in just a few more visits, when our son will achieve complete food freedom. This program is amazing and I encourage everyone I meet with food allergies to look into this program.

The Food Allergy Institute is a specialized clinic that focuses on the diagnosis, treatment, and management of food allergies. The clinic is located in the Long Beach, California area, and is headed by Dr. Inderpal Randhawa, who is a board-certified allergist and immunologist. They have recently added another clinic in San Diego.

The clinic provides a comprehensive evaluation of food allergies and utilizes cutting-edge diagnostic techniques to accurately diagnose food allergies. The clinic also offers individualized treatment plans for patients based on their specific food allergies, medical history, and other individual factors.

The clinic's treatment options include immunotherapy, such as oral immunotherapy (OIT) and sublingual immunotherapy (SLIT), as well as medication management, nutritional counseling, and ongoing monitoring of food allergy symptoms. In addition to clinical services, the Southern California Food Allergy Institute is also involved in research and education related to food allergies. The clinic participates in clinical trials and collaborates with other researchers to advance the field of food allergy treatment and management.

CHAPTER NINE

BEING AN ADVOCATE
FOR YOUR CHILD

As a parent of a child with food allergies, you are your child's most informed advocate. You know your child's allergies, symptoms, and triggers better than anyone else. It can be challenging to navigate the world of food allergies, but advocating for your child is essential to keep them safe and healthy.

One of the most critical aspects of advocating for your child is to never be afraid to ask questions. When you visit a doctor or allergist, be prepared with a list of questions to ask. If you do not understand something, speak up and ask for clarification. It is crucial to ensure that you understand your child's diagnosis and treatment plan fully.

Another essential aspect of advocating for your child is to never be afraid to stand up for them, but always be polite. When it comes to your child's safety, you cannot afford to be complacent or accommodating. Politely, yet firmly, communicate your child's food allergies and restrictions to those around you. Educate those who need it and set clear boundaries to keep your child safe.

It is essential to trust your instincts as a parent. No doctor is as motivated as you are to understand your child's food allergies. If something does not feel right, do not hesitate to seek a second opinion or request further testing. It is better to be overly cautious than to take unnecessary risks.

Remember, your child is not defined by their food allergies. While food allergies can be challenging, they are only one aspect of your child's life. It is important to focus on your child's strengths, talents, and interests. Encourage them to participate in activities that do not revolve around food, such as sports or art classes. Celebrate their accomplishments, big and small, and support them in all aspects of their life.

In conclusion, advocating for your food allergic child is critical to keep them safe and healthy. Be prepared to ask questions, stand up for your child, and trust your instincts. Remember that your child's food allergy is only one aspect of their life, and they are much more than their diagnosis. By working together, you can ensure that your child lives a happy, healthy, and fulfilling life.

CHAPTER TEN

KEEPING HOPE

Why do children suffer with life-threatening food allergies? What's the purpose, the reason, the big picture? Why does my son have to deal with this? Why does my whole family have to deal with this?

The 'why' questions can drive you straight to insanity if you linger there too long. The truth is that we may never know the reasons why our children are suffering from food allergies. The question we should ponder is what can we learn through this struggle. There are blessings in the trials. We just have to open our eyes to the blessings and stay out of the pit of anger.

"Finally, all of you, be like-minded, be sympathetic, love one another, be compassionate and humble." 1 Peter 3:8

One blessing our family has experienced is unity. Because one person cannot solely carry the weight of keeping our son safe, the entire family carries it together. We have become a team, a safety net woven together with love. Sometimes, it takes hardships to weave a beautiful tapestry.

We have learned to trust in God's plan. This is not an easy road. We traveled down the path of anger, sorrow, pleading for a cure, and even denial. We found dead ends at every one of those paths. God nudged us down the hard road of faith. He has been teaching us all along the way that we must trust in His plan. There is no other option that gives us peace. Anger, sorrow, denial all left us with turmoil inside. Faith, though it is sometimes difficult to keep, is the only road that leads to peace.

"For my thoughts are not your thoughts, neither are your ways may ways, declares the Lord." Isaiah 55:8

Looking at the blessings and focusing on gratefulness has left our family with more peace and encouragement than we could have imagined was possible at the beginning of this food allergy journey. We may not understand the whys of the weight we carry but what we can understand is the blessings. Focus on the positives, the gifts, and the blessings. You will see the world with a brighter light than before. This is my prayer for you-to seek the Lord in your trials and find your faith in Him.

"Rejoice in the Lord always. I will say it again: Rejoice! Let your graciousness be known to everyone. The Lord is near. Don't worry about anything, but in everything, through prayer and petition with thanksgiving, present your requests to God. And the peace of God, which surpasses all understanding, will guard your hearts and minds in Christ Jesus." Philippians 4: 4-7

Key Scripture Verses

1. "I can do all things through Christ who strengthens me." - Philippians 4:13

2. "Trust in the Lord with all your heart, and lean not on your own understanding; in all your ways acknowledge Him, and He will make your paths straight." - Proverbs 3:5-6

3. "The Lord is my strength and my shield; my heart trusts in him, and he helps me." - Psalm 28:7

4. "Do not be anxious about anything, but in every situation,

by prayer and petition, with thanksgiving, present your requests to God. And the peace of God, which transcends all understanding, will guard your hearts and your minds in Christ Jesus." - Philippians 4:6-7

5. "The Lord himself goes before you and will be with you; he will never leave you nor forsake you. Do not be afraid; do not be discouraged." - Deuteronomy 31:8

6. "But those who hope in the Lord will renew their strength. They will soar on wings like eagles; they will run and not grow weary, they will walk and not be faint." - Isaiah 40:31

7. "Come to me, all you who are weary and burdened, and I will give you rest." - Matthew 11:28

8. "For I am convinced that neither death nor life, neither angels nor demons, neither the present nor the future, nor any powers, neither height nor depth, nor anything else in all creation, will be able to separate us from the love of God that is in Christ Jesus our Lord." - Romans 8:38-39

9. "The Lord is my rock, my fortress and my deliverer; my God is my rock, in whom I take refuge, my shield and the horn of my salvation, my stronghold." - Psalm 18:2

10. "So do not fear, for I am with you; do not be dismayed, for I am your God. I will strengthen you and help you; I will uphold you with my righteous right hand." - Isaiah 41:10

CHAPTER ELEVEN

CONCLUDING THOUGHTS

My hope for every food allergy person and family is that you keep hope in your future. There is a plan for you and there are treatments available. Each year, there are more and more choices for allergy friendly foods, restaurants, and food-free activities. As we have navigated the world in the lens of food allergies, we have learned so much. It does become easier. The anxiety becomes manageable. There is an army of food allergy families there to support you and understand you. Food allergies have opened our entire families' eyes to all types of limiting medical conditions and the struggles people have to undergo. It has created empathy, understanding and a deep desire to help others. The silver lining is greater than the cloudy storm, though it may not seem that way as you are walking through it. There's beauty on the other side, you just need to look for it.

NOTES

RESOURCES

FARE (Food Allergy Research & Education) website: foodallergy.org

Spokin website: spokin.com

Food Allergy Institute website: foodallergyinstitute.com

Kids with Food Allergies website: kidswithfoodallergies.org

Red Sneakers for Oakley website: redsneakers.org

Elijah's Law: elijahalavifoundation.org

ACKNOWLEDGEMENT

Thank you to my son, Jaxon, for teaching me determination and perseverance. Without him, this resource would not exist. Putting my thoughts, research, and faith into words was therapeutic for me as a food allergy parent. I hope it helps you as much as it has me.

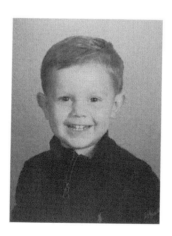

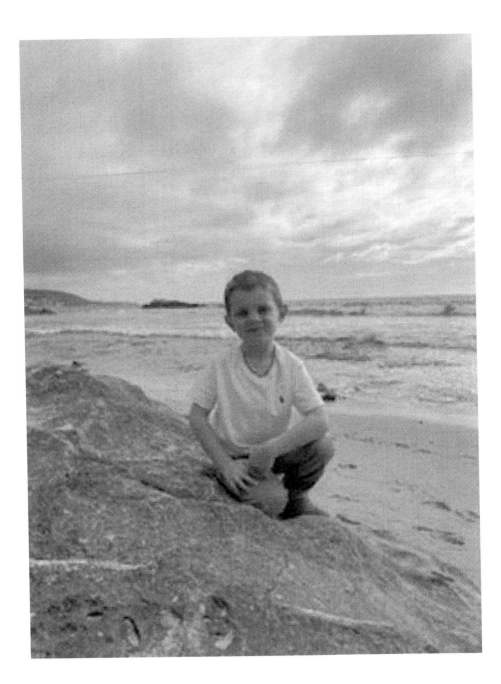

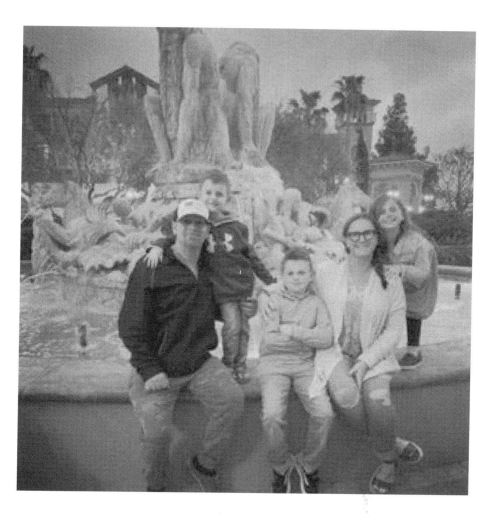

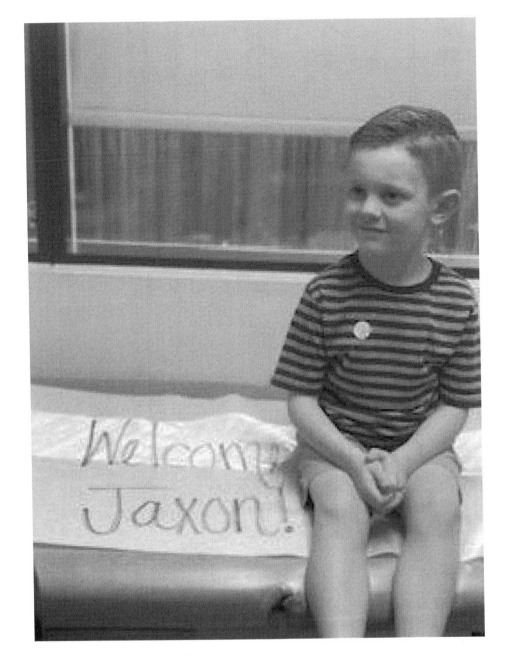

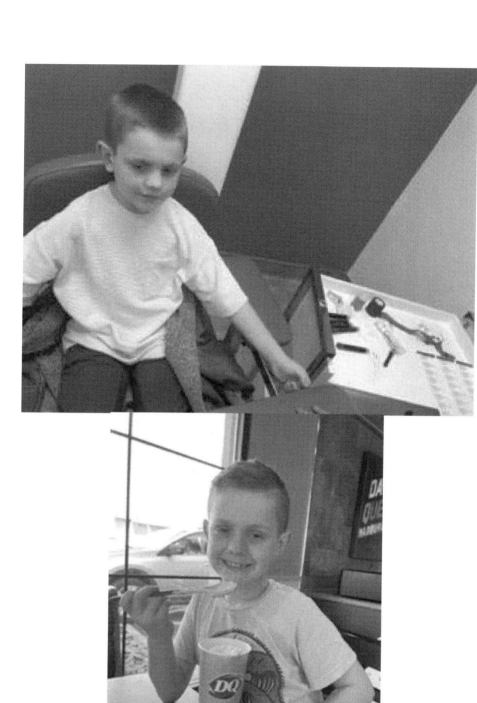

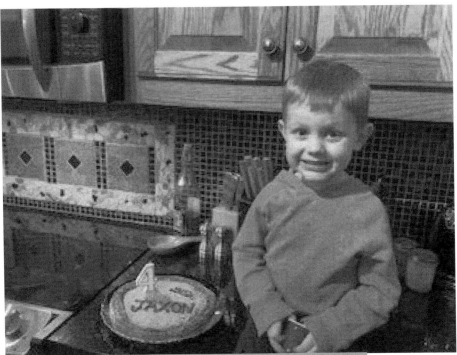

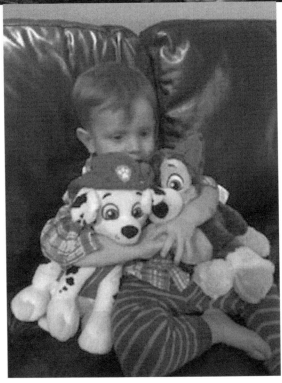

ABOUT THE AUTHOR

Melissa Cole

Melissa Cole, MA in Christian Ministry, is a food allergy parent and published devotional writer, featured in the Summer 2018 issue of The Secret Place. Melissa's writing has also been featured in The Liberty Leader newspaper and The Courier-Times newspaper . After learning of her son's life threatening food allergies when he turned one year old, she began researching everything food allergy related-treatment 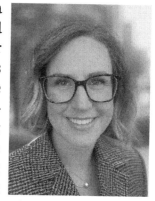 options, causes, coping strategies, recipes, and more. She found there were few resources available in print for new food allergy parents, so she embarked on the journey of writing "The Food Allergy Handbook" as a resource for parents, food allergy sufferers, and medical practitioners who want to learn more about food allergies, including the emotional side of food allergies.

PRAISE FOR AUTHOR

"The Food Allergy Handbook' is an essential compass, guiding you through the often challenging journey of food allergies. With its unique blend of practical advice, nourishing recipes, and heartfelt devotions, this book is a beacon of hope, making the complex world of food allergies more approachable and less intimidating."

- THOMAS SILVERA, CO-FOUNDER/VP OF THE ELIJAH-ALAVI FOUNDATION

PRAISE FOR AUTHOR

"To know what any journey is like, you listen to those who have walked the road before you. Melissa and her family have walked the path and now share the road with readers who are travelling the same road. Her words give hope and encouragement on a path that can seem lonely and overwhelming. There is light on this road, as evidenced by The Food Allergy Handbook. If you are walking this road, this handbook provides hope and resources. If someone you love is battling food allergies, grab this handbook and equip yourself to walk this road with them. I have watched Melissa and her family navigate life facing food allergies and have been inspired by their faith, perseverance, knowledge, and their resiliency."

- PASTOR ANDY CLAPP, AUTHOR OF "MIDNIGHT, CHRISTMAS EVE"

Made in the USA
Middletown, DE
25 October 2023

41254644R10046